Letter from the Pu

Amanda Klenner

Chocolate is a food that everyone knows and most people love, but did you know it has medicinal benefits? Cacao is one of those traditional ceremonial plants that has been distorted by our modern society from a sacred plant to a highly processed food that is overused, abused, and adulterated.

In Mayan culture, cacao (*Theobroma cacao*) was thought of as the "food of the gods" and was so highly valued that it was used as currency to pay taxes. When Europeans discovered cacao, they brought it back home with them, added milk and sugar, and created the chocolate we know and use today. Traditionally, however, it was used in an unsweetened form in sacred ceremonies to enhance trance-like states.

In the United States, we have taken cacao, cooked it, sugared it, added milk and call it cocoa. So when you hear someone call chocolate cocoa they generally are talking about the processed product, but when you hear them say cacao, they are talking about the plant and the raw plant materials.

Raw cacao has been touted as a super food in the natural health circles. I think after reading this issue you may get an idea as to why. Enjoy this with a nice cup of hot chocolate (home made herbal hot chocolate) or some delicious herbal cacao truffles and see just how cacao can benefit your body.

Green Blessings,

- *Amanda*

Table of Contents

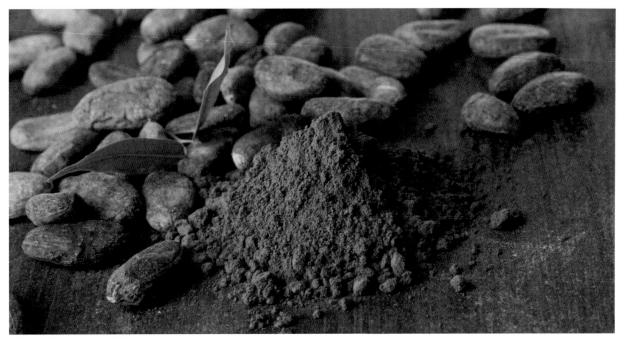

Cacao Herbal Monograph

Stephany Hoffelt

One of my fondest childhood memories is coming indoors on a cold winter day and waiting impatiently while Mom whipped up a batch of homemade hot cocoa. Our modern love affair with cocoa and chocolate go back to the days when the early Spanish and British explorers first brought it back from the New World. Although preparations and uses for the plant have changed over the centuries, the fact remains that cacao holds a special place in our culture. Few people stop to consider that what is now considered a confection was once widely used as a medicinal preparation. Cocoa powder and chocolate are both products that come from processing the cacao bean.

Scientific Name: *Theobroma cacao*

Family: Malvaceae

Other Names: cacao tree, cocoa tree

Origin of Cacao

The cacao tree is native to the Amazon Basin, but its range spread north to Central America when more cultures began cultivating it. The cacao tree will only flourish in very specific climatic conditions. It's a tropical undergrowth plant, and it depends upon high temperatures and humidity only found near the Equator. The trees also require the presence of the *Forcipomyia* midge, which inhabit these ecosystems, for pollination. Each of the roughly 12-inch (30 cm) pods growing from the trunk and main branches produce anywhere from 25 to 40 bitter-tasting seeds, or beans, which are surrounded by a white pulp. The beans are processed into powder, cocoa butter, and chocolate; the pulp is harvested for other uses. The pods will not open without some sort of mechanical assistance from animals or humans. Spider monkeys, who use the pods as a food source, earned the reputation as the "bringers of cacao" due to their efficient dispersal of the seeds.[1]

The Science

There are a lot of claims about cacao's superfood status, and even more traditional and modern suggested uses. I've included below a brief summary of what has been proven through scientific method.

Constituents

Cacao contains the xanthines theobromine and caffeine. It also contains the fatty acids stearic acid and oleic acid. Recent scientific research into the phenol content of chocolate has identified thousands of various polyphenols in chocolate including the flavonoid quercetin and the flavonols epicatechin and catechin.[2]

Actions

The theobromine in cacao acts as a central nervous system stimulant, working on both the cardiac and respiratory systems. Theobromine is also a diuretic, a vasodilator, and a smooth-muscle relaxant.[3] Caffeine is a central nervous system stimulant and diuretic too. Unlike theobromine, it is a vasoconstrictor.[4] It seems worth noting that these opposing actions of vasodilation and vasoconstriction could have a toning effect on the vasculature, although more research is needed to confirm this theory. The various phenolic compounds act as antioxidants and have anti-inflammatory actions, which contribute to cacao's positive "metabolic, antihypertensive, anti-inflammatory, and anti-thrombotic effects."[5] In addition to these actions, chocolate has been termed a euphoric, as it has been theorized to impact serotonin and endorphin levels in the brain.[6]

Cacaos Many Uses

Putting scientific method aside for a minute, there is an incredibly rich history of ethnobotanical use that continues up to the present day. While today cacao is thought of as food, historically cacao has been considered ceremonial, medicinal, and nutritive.

History and Tradition

Cacao's long history of both medicinal and ritual use began in Mesoamerica. The similarity between Aztec and Mayan use of the plant, point towards its use by a common ancestor.[7] According to both cultures, cacao was gifted to humans by the divine and was an integral part of religious rituals. The most common preparation was a drink made from cacao powder or paste cakes mixed with water. Depending on the area, the drinks contained additional ingredients such as chili powder, vanilla, or ground maize. The drink was typically frothed by making it in a special cacao pot with a spout for blowing into it, or by quickly transferring the drink between two vessels.[8]

Traditional cocoa powder preparations were considered to have antiseptic, diuretic, ecbolic (stimulating uterine contractions), emmenagogue, and parasiticide actions. Early Spanish explorers reported that indigenous peoples used cacao to treat angina, constipation, dental problems, dysentery, asthenia, gout, and many other diseases[9] including alopecia, burns, cough, dry lips, eyes, fever, diarrhea, listlessness, malaria, nephrosis, rheumatism, snakebite, and wounds.[10]

The use of cacao as a medicinal plant spread to Spain and Great Britain as these empires settled the Americas. In 1624, Spanish physician Santiago de Valverde Turices was the first to assign energetic qualities to both cacao powder and chocolate. He claimed that while the powder was cold, chocolate drinks were hot, dry, and suitable for cold, damp conditions.[11] Henry Stubbe was one of the first Europeans to write extensively on cacao. His text, titled *The Indian Nectar; or A discourse concerning chocolate wherein the nature of the cacao-nut is examined...*, was published in 1682. *Axtextli,* a beverage he mentioned as an aphrodisiac, was a mixture of cacao paste, maize, mecaxochitl (black pepper), and tlilxochitl (vanilla). In The *English American* published in 1648, Thomas Gage mentioned that black pepper mixed with cacao was a remedy for a "cold liver." *King's American Dispensatory* recommends a mixture of cacao and milk as a restorative drink for "persons convalescing from acute diseases." M. Grieves mentions in *A Modern Herbal* that in her time, cacao was given as a diuretic along with digitalis to relieve "accumulation of blood in the body resulting from cardiac failure" and as a remedy for hypertension due to the vasodilative action.

Modern Day

Although human studies of theobromine have confirmed its potential usefulness in inhibiting coughs,[12] for the most part, the use of cacao as a medicinal has faded out of practice. It is, however, still widely considered a dietary supplement with health-promoting qualities. There is a great deal of research available on the health benefits of adding cacao to our diets. The phenolic compounds seem to protect against chronic diseases related to oxidative stress, one study concluding, "Several in vivo studies have provided strong support for the hypothesis that the consumption of flavanol-rich foods, such as certain cocoas and chocolates, may be associated with reduced risk for vascular disease."[13] A study released last year has addressed the potential of cacao polyphenols in preventing "metabolic diseases and chronic inflammation associated with obesity."[14]

Since "milk proteins inhibit absorption of flavonoids" dark chocolate may be the best way to consume chocolate for the dietary benefits.[15] Cacao may also have mental health benefits. Ask many people, and they will tell you that they self-medicate on down days with chocolate. This practice seems to be supported by research on how eating chocolate impacts mood. Cocoa butter, which is another by-product of processing the beans, is used extensively in modern cosmetic preparations, due to its rich emollient properties, as well as in the chocolate-making process.

Using Cacao Safely

As with any food plant that is also a medicinal herb, there are some precautions to keep in mind as you incorporate it into your daily regimen.

Side Effects

Cacao can cause allergic reactions in some people, although that is rare, and it may trigger migraines in some individuals.[16] Many of its side effects are related to the caffeine content. As with all caffeinated beverages, moderation is key.

Contraindications and Drug Interactions

Avoid cacao if you have an allergy to any member of the *Sterculiaceae* family. People who suffer from kidney stones or gout may also want to avoid cacao as it increases urinary oxalate levels.[17]

There are a number of pharmaceutical drugs that interact with caffeine including clozapine, beta-adregenic antogonists, lithium, and drugs used for testing for heart conditions. Be sure to discuss your caffeine intake with your physician before starting a new prescription. The flavanols in cacao may also interact with blood-thinning medications.

Use During Pregnancy and Lactation

Follow your physician's recommendation regarding daily caffeine intake during pregnancy and while breastfeeding. In some studies, excessive caffeine in the maternal diet has resulted in colic in infants.[18]

Dosage and Administration

There are no established dosages for cacao powder. Administration is generally in the form of a beverage or confection. Half of a 3-ounce chocolate bar contains 86 – 240 mg of theobromine and 9 – 31 mg of caffeine.[19]

Cacao is a tasty and versatile herb. It is easy to incorporate into many recipes and you will rarely run across someone who objects to eating more chocolate. Around my home, cacao beverage blends are a handy way to mask other herbs that aren't as popular with the children. Have fun experimenting!

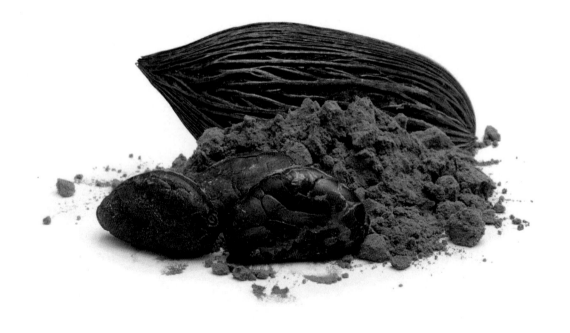

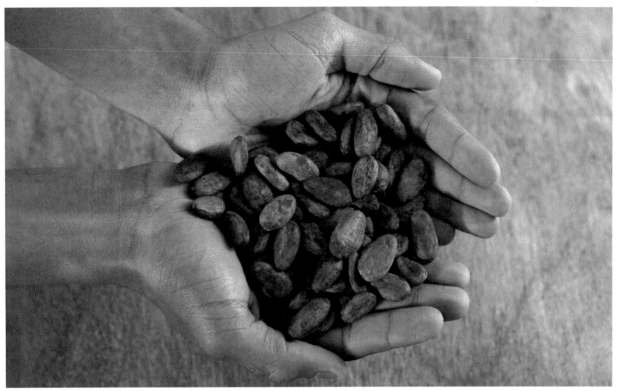

The Importance of Fair Trade

Heather Lanham

Cacao is beautiful, useful, tasty, and magical; but it has a darker side, and not just in the form of dark chocolate. Chocolate is big business, and it's now grown in many places. Unfortunately, Côte d'Ivoire is one of the places where the industry's dark side can be seen, in the form of child slavery. Côte d'Ivoire is the largest producer of cacao beans with current production approaching 2 million tons per year. The closest runner-up is Ghana, at just over a million tons.

The truth is, the vast majority of this cacao is picked via child labor. Legislation to end child labor in the chocolate fields was overwhelmingly blocked by the chocolate industry. According to UNICEF estimates from 2012, there were near half a million children working on the farms of Côte d'Ivoire. The legislation, having failed to pass, resulted only in a voluntary protocol.

Dark practices such as slave labor is why organizations like Fair Trade USA exist. They certify farmers, guaranteeing that they get a fair price for their crops, and that they are not participating in slave or child labor. I personally look for the Fair Trade labels on any cacao products I buy for my family. I sincerely hope that one day, Fair Trade certification won't be necessary.

So, when you chose to buy chocolate, be sure it is fair trade certified.

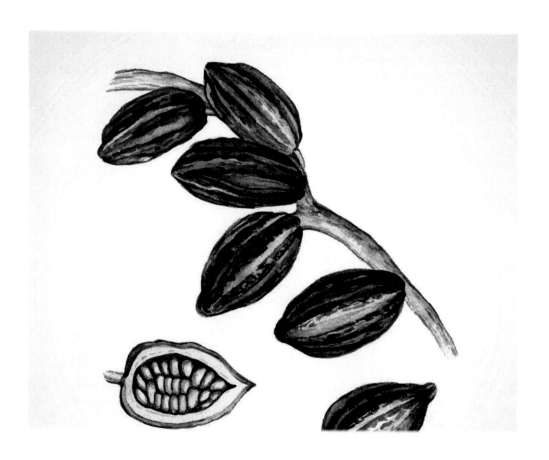

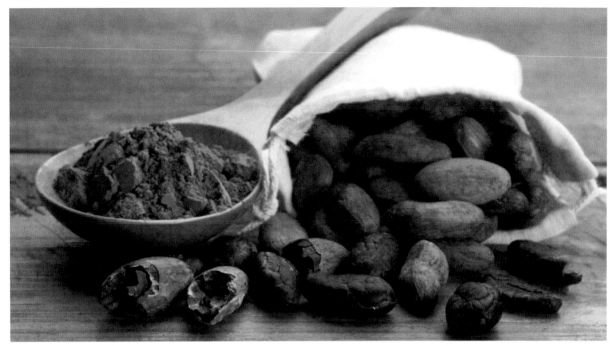

The Spiritual Heart of Cacao

Darcy Blue

I have been working with ceremonial cacao for three years in my practice as an herbalist and teacher, and though we all love chocolate for its sweetness and euphoric benefits, I have found that the medicine of cacao runs very deep into the soul realms as well.

Cacao is considered a strong medicine for the heart, with all its mineral, vitamin, and antioxidant constituents, and I consider it a powerful ally for the emotional and spiritual heart as well. Cacao seems to resonate with the energy of the heart chakra, allowing it to open and become more receptive to connection with another heart, or with the energy and wisdom of the soul.

I believe it also allows energy to flow more freely through the heart. If we think about the heart chakra (the physical heart and the emotional heart) we can easily recognize it as a center place within the physical and spiritual energetic levels of the body. It is actually the hub, or crucible, of energies and impulses which come to us through the earth and into the lower chakras, as well as the energies that come down from the heavens, and through our upper chakras—they meet in the heart center. It is literally and figuratively a container and director for these energies in the body.

A well-functioning heart chakra is absolutely vital for a fully realized and satisfying life. If we operate only from our physical needs, ego, and lower chakras, we can become selfish, stagnant, and cut off from our higher development as a human. Likewise, if we only or primarily operate from the upper chakras, seeking complete detachment from our humanity, we may become spaced-out, disconnected from physical reality and human experience. We need to be able to channel and work with both through the heart to be fully human in this life, to be balanced between our spiritual growth and tending to our physical body and its needs.

Cacao has this affinity to the spiritual development of the heart chakra energetically, while also being a medicine that stimulates physical stamina and energy. It also possesses mild entheogenic (shamanic) properties that alter our mood, brain chemistry, and perception of reality.

I semi-regularly offer ceremonial cacao in my community, as an opportunity for people to work with the stronger form of cacao as a spiritual medicine. These experiences are always guided toward helping people to connect more deeply with their hearts. Our culture is one that devalues the wisdom of the heart, and I believe we can benefit from working with medicines that help us (as individuals and as a culture) to reconnect with the power of our own heart wisdom.

When we open our hearts through the use of a stimulating dose of cacao, we more easily access the energies running through the hub and find balance between our physical and spiritual needs. Our perception opens to become more available to hear what the heart is trying to tell us. This can cover a range of purposes: healing work for recovery from grief or heartache, creative inspirations that take us closer to living our soul's purpose, or learning to cultivate a healthier, more loving, authentic, and compassionate connection with the people in our lives. I use shamanic journey and guided meditation to bring people into a place where they can access their own heart personally. Shamanic dance, Journey Dance, and creative expression are all great ways to help deliver cacao medicine to the heart.

Cacao is a wonderful and friendly ally for the heart in less serious ceremonial moments too, like when we need to invite heart-to-heart connections with people in our lives; or when our heart is grieving and needs fortification and strengthening. Cacao is also known as a remedy for the blues, and many people eat chocolate when they are feeling sad, moody, or low. I also like to include cacao in strengthening teas for the emotional heart with rose, hawthorn, and other heart remedies. Drinking a small cup of rich raw cacao drink (not a strong ceremonial dose) can be used similarly to connect us with the heart chakra, our creative impulses, our sexuality, and our compassionate nature. Cacao is considered by many to be food for the heart, on a physical level, and I also think of it as spiritual food for the heart.

A symbol and energy of abundance, cacao was used in traditional cultures as a currency and as an offering to royalty. I often call upon this abundant quality of cacao medicine when I feel disconnected from the flow of financial plenty, or when I want to manifest resources for a new endeavor. I like to use whole raw cacao beans on my altar, or in energetic medicine bundles and pouches worn around the neck. We can rub the beans gently to remind us to connect with abundance and flow and allow ourselves to receive it.

Cacao is rich, abundant, and desirable. We crave chocolate, and the sweetness it offers us. It is important, however, to connect with the whole plant medicine of cacao, before processing and diluting it—taste its bitterness, strength, and richness. I even like to think of bitter cacao as a medicine for a bitter heart, restoring openness, love, resilience, strength, abundance of feeling, and the ability to receive love.

Ceremonial Cacao Drink

Traditionally, cacao has been served strong, dark, and unsweetened as a ceremonial drink to enhance creativity, spiritual awareness, physical stamina, heart opening, and as an aphrodisiac. Drinking cacao in this fashion is a far cry from our more familiar beverage, highly sweetened and diluted with milk, and is a much more powerful and medicinally active form of cacao to work with.

Note that the strong dose can be a bit much for the stomach at first. Starting with smaller doses and working up to a bigger dose is wise. Also remember that the effects of cacao taken in this way last for 5-6 hours, and you may find yourself with lots of extra energy, in a giddy mood, or feeling particularly open and heady. Please be sure to provide yourself a safe, nurturing, creative environment to use the time well. I encourage people to engage in a creative activity during this time, dance or do yoga, or explore some deep journey work, meditation, or journaling. Sleeplessness is a common side effect of high doses of cacao. Some people may experience mild stomach upset. Or, you may just find yourself blissed out!

Ingredients

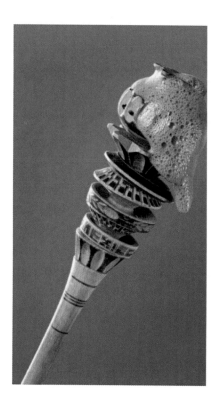

- 1–2 ounces cacao paste or finely ground beans per person (my favorite to use is Heartblood Cacao)
- 8 ounces boiling water (or a strong infusion of an herb like rose, lavender, marigold, or tulsi)
- 1–2 tsp cinnamon powder
- 1 Tbsp vanilla extract
- 1/16 tsp cayenne powder
- 1/8 tsp sea salt
- 2 pinches freshly ground nutmeg
- honey to taste

Directions

1. Melt the cacao paste into hot water or tea, and whisk it well.
2. Whisk in the spices just before serving.
3. You may wish to sweeten this drink if you are unfamiliar with bitter cacao, as it is quite strong. If you would like to dilute it further for less intensity, you can use a bit of cream or coconut milk. I occasionally also like to add 1–2 Tbsp of organic corn masa flour (masa harina) to my cacao when whisking for a heartier, more warming drink.
4. Drink slowly over 30 minutes to allow the medicine of cacao to take effect. You may wish to have a light snack available after sipping the cacao, but it is stronger when taken on an empty stomach.

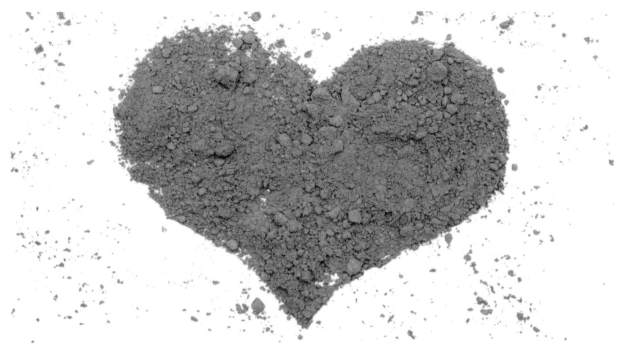

Cacao for the Heart

Stephany Hoffelt

Modern research on the health benefits of cacao frequently focus on its cardiovascular health effects. The first time these benefits were noted was in a study of the Kuna Indians, which concluded that their daily intake of unprocessed cacao kept them from developing age-related cardiovascular deterioration.[1]

There are many types of disorders affecting the cardiovascular system, some natural consequences of aging. Arterial stiffness occurs due, in part, to reduced collagen production as we age. In working with elders, I frequently see a wide pulse pressure—the systolic blood pressure is quite high, while the diastolic reading is pretty low. Physicians call this *isolated systolic hypertension*, and it occurs due to reduced distensibility of the aorta.

Other disorders, on the other hand, are results of lifestyle habits such as unhealthy diet, lack of exercise, or poor stress management. These factors contribute to systemic inflammation, which is the root cause of many diseases, including atherosclerosis (buildup of plaque on the artery walls). The process by which atherosclerosis occurs is as follows: During the inflammation response, various cells (such as smooth muscle cells, monocytes, and lymphocytes) migrate to damaged areas to help repair them, adhering to the endothelium (inner lining of the blood vessels). This results in a fibrous lesion, which in turn distends the artery. If the cause of the inflammation is not resolved, these lesions grow, blocking the flow of blood and trapping large molecules such as LDL cholesterol.

Small arteries in the body are the first to become plugged, which may lead to problems such as numbness in the feet and hands as peripheral circulation becomes impaired, or erectile dysfunction in men. The problem then moves on to larger arteries in the body and ultimately may lead to *coronary artery disease* (CAD). Early warning signs of CAD include chest pain upon exertion, shortness of breath, and fatigue. Your body may also compensate for poor lifestyle habits by raising your blood pressure, but little is known about the direct mechanism that causes the blood pressure to elevate.

Adding cacao to your diet, along with making necessary lifestyle improvements, can help to improve cardiovascular function and mitigate the damage caused by chronic inflammation. The reason for this has to do with how constituents of cacao modulate inflammation. Cardiovascular disease activates pro-inflammatory enzymes in the body. The phenolic compounds in cacao liqueur stimulate nitric oxide production, which reduces the impact of inflammatory enzymes on the body by suppressing production of pro-inflammatory cytokines.[2] The procyanidins present in cacao also increase the production of anti-inflammatory cytokines.[3]

Cacao Elixirs

When I began making elixirs, I saw these preparations as a good way to get cacao into my daily diet, without the added fats and sugars that are present in hot chocolate beverages or candy bars. While this magazine issue focuses on the benefits of *Theobroma cacao*, I would be remiss if I did not mention a few other herbs that could be incorporated into your elixir formulas, which would increase their efficacy as heart tonics. Modern research supports the use of berberine, a constituent of the *Berberis* genus of plants, in mobilizing endothelial progenitor cells, which ultimately improves the elasticity of small arteries.[4] Other studies support the use of hawthorn in lowering systolic blood pressure.[5]

I like to make my cacao elixirs with a base of cacao and hawthorn, adding *corrigents* that I think are appropriate to the constitution of the person who will be enjoying the elixir. *Corrigent* is a fancy word for a flavoring agent. Clearly though, these herbs lend their own action to a formula. When formulating, I like to give some thought to these actions. Most types of pepper, for example, act to stimulate blood flow to peripheral parts of the body; but keep in mind that cayenne can be too drying for some people, especially elders. Indian Long Pepper (*Piper longum*) is a less drying alternative. Orange peel contributes more flavonoids to a formula, improves digestion, and is mildly warming. Nutmeg in very small doses has been shown to have anxiolytic (anti-anxiety) properties.[6] Cinnamon helps the body to regulate glucose levels.

I like to start with two parts cacao nibs to one part dried hawthorn berries and then toss things in based on intuition. The following are two formulas that I have found particularly tasty.

Ingredients

- 2 parts cacao nibs
- 1 part dried hawthorn berries
- 1/4 part dried orange peels
- 1/8 part freshly grated nutmeg
- Honey to taste

OR

- 2 parts cacao nibs
- 1 part hawthorn
- 1/4 part tart cherries
- 1/8 part cayenne
- Honey to taste

Directions

1. Place herbs in an appropriate sized mason jar.
2. Add honey.
3. Pour brandy over the contents until it completely covers all the herbal material. I like Laird's Apple Brandy because it is a higher proof and I think it cuts the soapy flavor of the hawthorn a little.

4. After 4 weeks, strain the herbs out of the honey-brandy mix. A tincture press is really handy here, but if you don't have one, you can strain with a cheese cloth, strainer, and funnel. You can use a potato ricer to squeeze even more goodness out of the plant material after that, but this is optional.

5. Store in a dark place or in amber jars to protect your elixir from light so it lasts longer and stays potent.

6. Enjoy perhaps a tablespoon or so mixed into another beverage or by itself once a day.

You can obviously come up with infinite blends of your own. I've made a chocolate-mint blend before, and a coffee-cacao elixir. Both were thoroughly enjoyed by their consumers. Whatever flavor you choose, you can sip these elixirs straight, from a small cordial glass, or as alternative to honey in flavoring an herbal infusion. I like to use elixirs to perk up bland infusions such as oatstraw. These beverages are mildly stimulating due to the caffeine and I have had a few clients who enjoy them as a morning pick-me-up. You are only limited by your imagination in the combinations that you put together, and you know best what you enjoy. So have fun with the preparations and enjoy your tonic elixirs regularly!

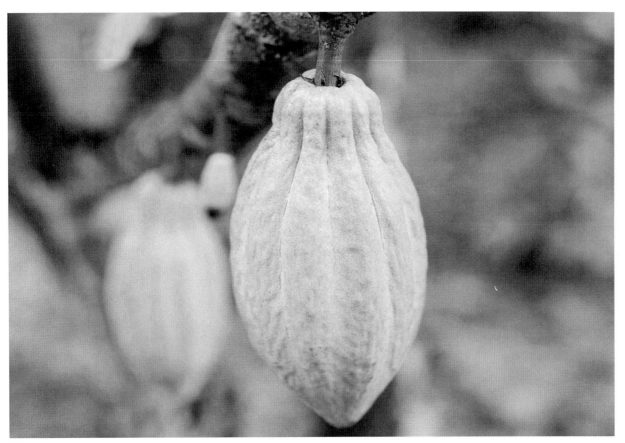

The Flesh of Madre Cacao

Jessica Morgan

Cacao evokes warmth, comfort, and passion, doesn't it? Usually sweet passion. Many say that just thinking about cacao can evoke a pleasurable response. We crave it. But we crave lots of sensory feelings from things like music, aromatic smells, sultry tastes; because all of these senses bring out deep desires in us. Perhaps it's the nature of the tree that gives chocolate some of its intense, exotic taste and pleasurable qualities. The cacao trees flourish in the hot, drizzly, humid belt of the Equator sheltered within the understory of the noisy evergreen rainforest. Their nature is hot, humid and energetically a lot like our passion-filled selves.

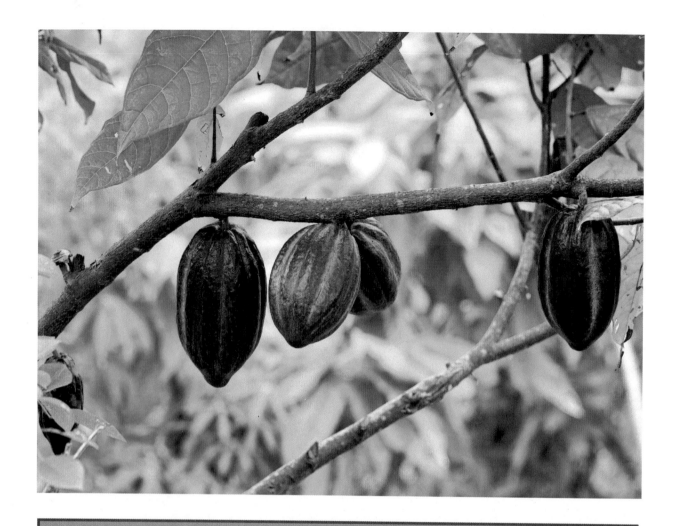

All you need is love. But a little chocolate now and then doesn't hurt. ~Charles M. Schulz

I was blessed to spend some time with the cacao tree last year during one of my herbal immersion weekends with Heidi Jarvis from the School of Natural Medicine at the Denver Botanic Gardens. I think the ability to commune with nature is embedded deep within us, and we don't have to be in the depths of the wilderness to enjoy it; a tree in our backyard or in a greenhouse, or even a little houseplant in a pot has something to say.

We sat with a lot of different medicine plants and trees that day, but the time spent in the greenhouse with the cacao tree was truly ripening. It was hot, steamy and wet....a lot like the bedroom! And as we sat to commune with the tree, there was this feeling of nourishment and excitement. It was both stimulating and relaxing at the same time. It's a very loving tree with a bewitching nature. Just her presence makes you feel loved. She reminded me to love myself, to be strong with self-reliance, to keep connection between women, and that when we nurture ourselves, we can then nurture others.

Cacao's tastes and smells strengthen the light body and etheric endorphins, leading to feelings of euphoria, the release of sex hormones, and a sense of spiritual wellbeing. (*Etheric endorphins* refers to the human energy field, and can be thought of as a kind of aura, or "good vibrations.")

The cacao tree, which is also known as Madre Cacao, would be fairly easy to grow if you were to provide her with the right environment. You would just need to live in a tropical climate, or have the ability to grow the plant indoors, preferably in a giant shady and humid greenhouse.

Cacao is a relatively small tree with deeply gnarled bark and a twisting trunk that reaches out at you to showcase her glorious, gourd-shaped fruit pods. And, when you split open her fruit, you'll find cacao seeds encased in a sort of gooey, mucilaginous white pulp, called "baba de cacao" in South America. From the seeds come the beloved cacao powder and cacao butter.

After the beans are harvested, they're fermented, dried, roasted, and pressed. This process releases the vegetable fat from the beans, which we know as cocoa butter. Comprising a combination of edible saturated fats that are solid at room temperature but liquid at human body temperature, cocoa butter is the reason that chocolate literally melts in your mouth. It's used to make lip balms and salves, lotions, and pharmaceuticals like suppositories. Using cocoa butter topically on the skin is a treat like no other—it smells divine and leaves your skin glowing, vibrant, revitalized, soft, and supple. Taste it, smell it, feel it on your skin. It's euphoria for your senses!

Cocoa Butter vs Cacao Butter

Cacao butter is the pure, cold-pressed oil of the cacao bean. Raw cacao butter production doesn't exceed 115°F (46°C), while cocoa butter might undergo more heating during the pressing process. Raw cacao butter is more nutrient-dense, but otherwise, they are fully interchangeable. Both are edible, stable vegetable fats that can be used in cooking and in preparations of skin and beauty products.

Cocoa butter is available in two forms—unrefined or refined. The differences are as follows:

- Unrefined: Unrefined cocoa butter is simply cocoa butter in its unprocessed form. It's a creamy yellow color and smells just like chocolate.
- Refined: Refined cocoa butter is stripped of its scent and color, making it suitable for herbals and cosmetic recipes where one does not want a product with an aroma of chocolate. However, heavy processing to eliminate color and scent also strips the healing property of the product itself.

As I've said, cocoa butter melts at body temperature, and if we gently warming it in the palms of our hands and then glide it onto skin, it becomes a wonderful massage oil. It also makes an excellent addition to products like lip balms and body butters for this same reason. Below is a recipe for one of my favorite body butters to nourish the skin for ourselves and our lovers. It's a gift from the flesh of the beautiful Madre Cacao. Enjoy!

Bedroom Body Dessert

Cacao's butter is the key ingredient that gives chocolate that yummy, creamy, and satisfying melt-in-your-mouth quality, and it will do the same on your skin. Body Dessert is an edible cacao butter, coconut butter, and vanilla bean kissing and licking balm, and it's good enough to eat! It's a simple delight for all you wild lovers out there. Massage this organic and orgasmic body dessert balm anywhere you want to kiss or be kissed. It could very easily be scooped into a cup of coffee or stirred into some porridge too, but it's much better as a kissing balm!

Ingredients
- 1/4 C organic raw cacao butter
- 1/4 C organic coconut butter

- 1/4 C organic unrefined virgin coconut oil
- 1/2 tsp vanilla bean extract
- Seeds from 1/2 vanilla bean

Directions

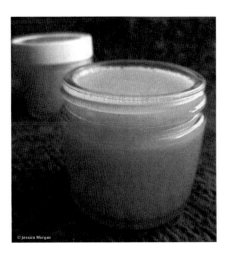

1. Scoop butters, oils, and vanilla into a double boiler and gently melt the ingredients together.
2. Once blended, pour the mix into a pretty jar and allow it to cool.
3. Enjoy! This body dessert makes a wonderful sensual massage balm and is safe for breasts, nipples, lips, and other personal areas.

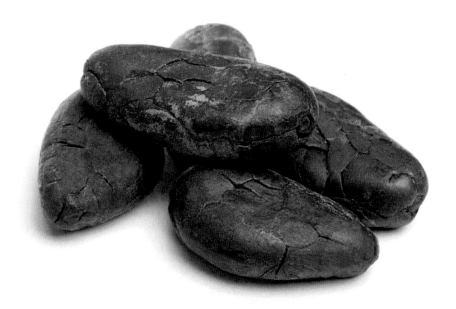

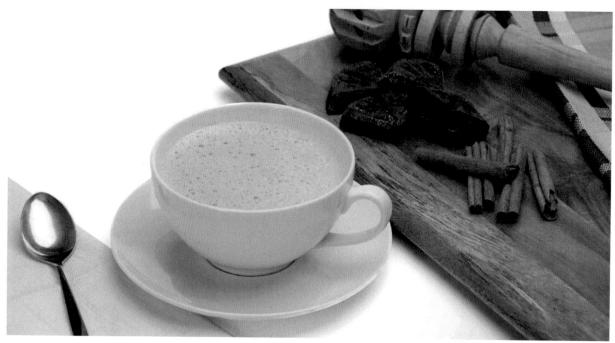

My Favorite Cacao Recipes

Amanda Klenner

In Jessica's article "The Flesh of Madre Cacao," she talks about what cocoa butter is, what it's used for, and some luscious and decadent uses for it. In this article, I will share some of my favorite uses for cacao in its many forms. For example, I often use cocoa butter in body butters, lip balms, salves, and so much more. I also have started incorporating cocoa powder into some bath and body care products, but I mostly reserve that precious stuff for eating.

Body Care Recipes

Many of the body care recipes here can be modified by adding a few drops of essential oils or by changing the other carrier oils to something you prefer to work with. If you are subbing for oils, be sure to choose an oil with a similar texture: solid oils (like palm) in place of coconut oil, or other liquid oils (like almond, avocado, or jojoba) instead of olive oil. This way, your recipe should still maintain the correct consistency. You can also, in most cases, substitute some part of the cocoa butter with shea butter to get a creamier consistency. Have fun playing with these delicious recipes!

Cocoa-licious Body Butter

When I first started making my own body care products, it was really just to reduce the chemical load I was putting on my body. Little did I know how simple and luxurious homemade bath and body care could be. I absolutely love this easy body butter. Not only does it whip up beautifully, but it smells delightful and can be dressed up however you like. The ingredients couldn't be simpler, more natural, or better for your skin. I often have people say that it smells good enough to eat! I wouldn't recommend it though: Dad tried it and said it isn't nearly as tasty as it looks (although it isn't harmful).

Ingredients

- 1 C cocoa butter
- 1/2 C coconut oil
- 1/2 C herb-infused oil (I love calendula-infused olive oil, but you can use almond, jojoba, olive, meadow foam, or any combination of oils you like)
- 10-15 drops essential oils of your choice (completely optional, but mint is always a delicious addition to cocoa)

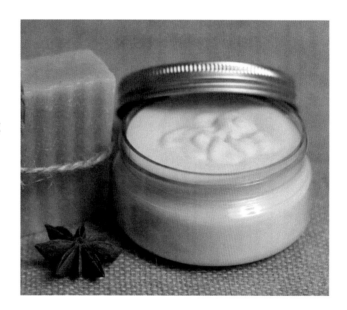

Directions

1. Melt the cocoa butter and coconut oil together using the double-boiler method in a large Pyrex bowl.
2. Once they are completely melted together, remove the mixture from the heat.
3. Add the olive oil and essential oils.
4. Let it sit until it cools. In the winter, letting it sit outside is the fastest way for it to cool down. (If you plan to use a hand mixer with a whisk, do not let it solidify completely. Rather, start to mix it as soon as a hardened layer forms on the sides of the bowl. If you're using a stand mixer or hand beaters you can wait until it is cooled to almost solid.)

5. Beat the oil mixture until it turns white and forms peaks.

6. Put the butter into a container of your choice and enjoy the luxurious moisturizing power of this great body butter!

This recipe makes about enough body butter to fill one 20-ounce flip-top container.

Lotion Bar Base Recipe

Sometimes we just need a little extra skin love that is long-lasting and adds a bit of protection to the skin. As long as you don't live somewhere hot, this bar is perfect to keep with you and moisturize as you go. These are so easy to make, and they take a lot less time than the body butter. In fact, if you don't have a good mixer, this might be a better option to enjoy the cocoa buttery goodness.

Ingredients

- 1/2 C coconut oil, infused with calendula flowers
- 1/2 C cocoa butter
- 1/2 C beeswax (grated or pastilles)
- Optional: essential oils that you enjoy

Directions

1. Melt coconut oil, cocoa butter, and beeswax using the double-boiler method in a pourable Pyrex dish.

2. Once the contents are completely melted, remove it from the heat.

3. Add 10-15 drops of your essential oil(s).

4. Pour the mixture into individual containers (preferably silicone molds, because it's easy to pop the bars out of them without any sticking).

5. Let cool until solid.

6. Use whenever you feel the need for a little extra moisture!

Note: Store these bars below 77°F, or they might melt.

Cocoa-Coffee Sugar Scrub

Did you ever want to just wake up and rub yourself all over with coffee and chocolate? No? Well you will now! This moisturizing, invigorating, and tissue-toning body scrub will exfoliate, encourage circulation to the skin, and help reduce cellulite. Also, chocolate and coffee! You're welcome. (This makes a great gift too!)

Ingredients

- 1 C ground coffee
- 1 C sugar
- 1/2 C cocoa powder
- 3 Tbsp olive or jojoba oil
- 2 Tbsp raw honey
- 10-30 drops of essential oils, depending on how strong you like the smell

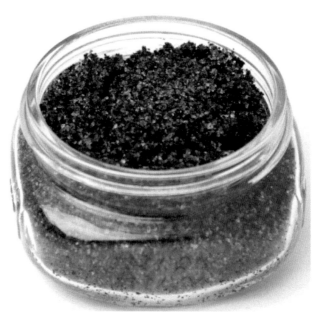

Directions

1. Combine the ingredients in a mixing bowl until thoroughly mixed.

2. The texture you are looking for is moist sticky grains. You do not want it to be too runny (add 1 Tbsp sugar until the right texture) or too dry (add 1 Tsp olive oil until the right texture).

3. Be sure the honey is incorporated into the mix.

4. Place in jars and enjoy!

5. Use in the shower after washing and shaving as a scrub to remove dry skin, reduce cellulite, and revitalize body and mind.

Lip Balm

The cost of lip balm in grocery stores is outrageous. Five dollars for a half-ounce tube of lip balm? No thank you! I can make my own delicious, natural, and tasty lip balm for under one dollar per tube or tin. What could be better?

Ingredients

- 1 Tbsp coconut oil
- 1 Tbsp beeswax
- 1 Tbsp cocoa butter
- 2 drops peppermint or spearmint essential oil (optional)
- 2 drops lavender essential oil (optional)

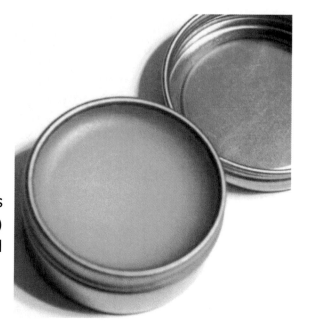

Directions

1. In a double boiler, melt all oils together (except the essential oils) on low heat until they're well blended.
2. Remove from heat.
3. Add essential oils and stir.
4. Pour into lip balm tubes or tins.
5. Let the containers cool and harden for 10-15 minutes before capping.

Consumable Recipes

The following recipes are every bit as decadent as the body care recipes above, and they're edible!

Homemade Cocoa Hazelnut Spread

You know that super-popular chocolate hazelnut spread you can get from the grocery store? The one that starts with nut and ends with ella? Well, if you don't, you are missing out on some delicious goodness! Unfortunately, the ingredients in the name-brand spread leave a lot to be desired in the "real food" department (although its not nearly as bad as it could be). Here is my knock-off recipe with real-food ingredients. As a bonus, this recipe is dairy-free, which the original spread is not.

Warning! You may find this spread ends up on a lot of foods that otherwise would have gone without an additional chocolaty topping like brownies, cookies, fingers, bananas, apples, ice cream, sandwiches, crackers, and so much more.

Ingredients

- 2 C raw hazelnuts
- 1 Tbsp vanilla extract
- 1/3 C cocoa powder
- 1/4 – 1/3 C sugar
- 1/4 tsp salt
- 2 tsp oil
- 1/2 C coconut milk

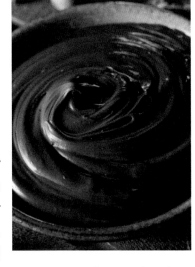

Notes: I use coconut sugar or turbinado sugar for this recipe, but some people use maple syrup and xylitol in a recipe similar to this with great results. I use almond, peanut, or coconut oil. This is an optional addition that helps make the spread extra creamy, but it's perfectly good without the extra oil! And finally, you can use any milk you like, but I think coconut milk is best in this recipe.

Directions

1. Roast your hazelnuts on a flat baking sheet at 400°F for 6–8 minutes.
2. Rub them together briskly in a dry paper towel until the skins come off. If you have a few stragglers with skin still on them, it isn't the end of the world.

3. In a high-powered blender or food processor, add the hazelnuts and blend them until they become a nut butter. If it looks chunky, keep blending. It can take up to 10 minutes to reach the right consistency.

4. Add the oil here if you would like the butter to be creamier.

5. Once the hazelnuts are the right consistency, add the additional ingredients.

6. Blend well, and enjoy!

Note: Be sure to keep this refrigerated. The milk makes it perishable, so enjoy it within a few weeks.

Kid-Friendly Hot Chocolate

Darcy shared with us a beautiful ceremonial cacao recipe, but I wanted to share a more family-friendly version of this sweet drink we all know and love. Now, you may think making your own hot cocoa from scratch is difficult, but my four-year-old can make this without my help (and tries when I'm not looking, little ninja that she is).

This recipe is easily modifiable for those with food intolerances or allergies. Traditional, vegan, or paleo, this recipe is easy to customize to fit your family's eating habits. Use more or less sugar and cacao powder to taste.

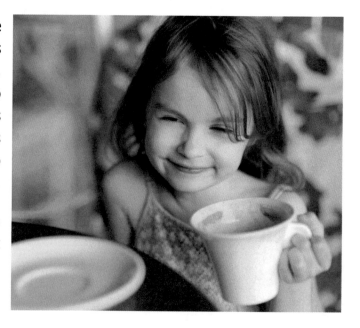

This recipe makes two 1-cup servings. If you want more, just double the recipe!

Ingredients
- 2 C milk of your choice (e.g., cow, coconut, almond, hemp seed, or any other)

- 2 Tbsp sweetener (e.g., honey, raw sugar, maple syrup, coconut sugar)
- 1/4 C cacao powder
- 1 tsp vanilla extract (or more if you like)
- Herbs of choice (optional)

Notes: You can use cacao powder, or the heated and processed Dutch cocoa, which is easy to find at the store and has similar health benefits. The herbs are optional. Adding a little aromatic spice or herb can bring a wonderful health boost as well as some fun flavor. Some herbs we add are ginger, cinnamon, rosemary, turmeric, peppermint, nutmeg, cardamom, rose, etc.

Directions

1. Pop all your ingredients into a non-reactive pan (I use stainless steel) and warm it up enough to enjoy a nice hot drink, but not above 120 degrees (or you lose some of those health benefits of raw cacao and honey).
2. With a handheld mixer or whisk, whip up the drink so it has a nice froth.
3. Enjoy!

Note: If you're using sugar instead of honey or maple syrup as a sweetener, you can make this in large batches to be used whenever you're ready for a delicious treat!

References

Cacao Herbal Monograph

Nisao Ogata, Arturo Gómez-Pompa, and Karl A. Taube, "The Domestication and Distribution of Theobroma cacao L. in the Neotropics," *Chocolate in Mesoamerica: A Cultural History of Cacao* ed. Cameron L. McNeil (University Press of Florida: Gainesville, 2006), 87.

[2] Chiaki Sanbongi, Naomi Osakabe, et al., "Antioxidative Polyphenols Isolated from Theobroma cacao," *Journal of Agricultural and Food Chemistry* 46, (1998). Abstract only: http://www.ncbi.nlm.nih.gov/pubmed/10554262

[3] Lisa Ganora, *Herbal Constituents*, (Herbalchem Press, 2009), 155.

[4] Ibid.

[5] G. Lippi, M. Franchini, et al., "Dark chocolate: consumption for pleasure or therapy?" *Journal of Thrombosis Thrombolysis* 28, (2013). Abstract only: http://www.ncbi.nlm.nih.gov/pubmed/18827977

[6] Gordon Parker, Isabella Parker, and Heather Brotchie, "Mood state effects of chocolate," *Journal of Affective Disorders* 92 (2006). Summary: http://www.blackdoginstitute.org.au/docs/Chocolatearticlesummary.pdf

[7] "Caroline Seawright. Life Death and Chocolate in Mesoamerica," (archaeological essay, 2012). Full text: http://www.thekeep.org/~kunoichi/kunoichi/themestream/ARC2AZT, 13.

[8] Hillary Christopher, "Cacao's Relationship with Mesoamerican Society." *Spectrum* 3, (2012). Full text: http://cola.unh.edu/sites/cola.unh.edu/files/student-journals/5_SPECTRUM_Christopher.pdf

[9] Donatella Lippi, "Chocolate and medicine: Dangerous liaisons?" *Nutrition* 25, (2009). Abstract only: http://www.ncbi.nlm.nih.gov/pubmed/19818277

[10] "Chocolate," National Standard Food, Herbs and Supplements Database (2014)

[11] Lippi, "Dangerous liasons."

[12] OS Usmani, MG Belvisi, et al., "Theobromine inhibits sensory nerve activation and cough." *The Journal of the Federation of American Studies for Experimental Biology* 19 (2005). Full text: http://www.fasebj.org/content/early/2005/01/27/fj.04-1990fje.long

[13] Carl Keen, Roberta Holt, "Cocoa Antioxidants and cardiovascular health," *American Journal of Clinical Nutrition* 81, (2005). Full text: http://ajcn.nutrition.org/content/81/1/298S.long

[14] Faisal Ali, Amin Ismail, and Sander Kersten. "Molecular mechanisms underlying the potention antiobesity-related diseases effect of cocoa polyphenols *Molecular Nutrition Food Research* 00 (2013). Abstract only: http://www.ncbi.nlm.nih.gov/pubmed/24259381

[15] G. Lippi, M. Franchini, et al. "Dark chocolate: consumption for pleasure or therapy?" *Journal of Thrombosis Thrombolysis* 28, (2013).

The Importance of Fair Trade

David McKenzie, Brent Swails, "Child slavery and chocolate: All too easy to find," *The CNN Freedom Project* January 19, 2012. http://thecnnfreedomproject.blogs.cnn.com/2012/01/19/child-slavery-and-chocolate-all-too-easy-to-find/

David McKenzie, "How to help: Slavery in the supply chain," *The CNN Freedom Project* January 17, 2012. http://thecnnfreedomproject.blogs.cnn.com/2012/01/17/how-to-help-slavery-in-the-supply-chain-2/

"Production - Latest figures from the Quarterly Bulletin of Cocoa Statistics," International Cocoa Organization. http://www.icco.org/about-us/international-cocoa-agreements/cat_view/30-related-documents/46-statistics-production.html

"Products: Cacao," Fair Trade USA. http://fairtradeusa.org/products-partners/cocoa

Cacao for the Heart

[1] Davide Grassi, Claudio Ferrie, "Cocoa, Flavonoids and Cardiovascular Protection," *Polyphenols in Human Health and Disease* Vol. 2, (Academic Press, 2013).

[2] Robert Corti, et al., "Cocoa and cardiovascular health," *Circulation* 119 (2009). Full text:
http://circ.ahajournals.org/cgi/pmidlookup?view=long&pmid=19289648

[3] Carl Keen, Roberta Holt, "Cocoa antioxidants and cardiovascular health" *American Journal of Clinical Nutrition* 81, (2005). Full text:
http://ajcn.nutrition.org/content/81/1/298S.long

[4] MG Xu, et al., "Berberine-induced mobilization of circulating endothelial progenitor cells improves human small artery elasticity," *Journal of Human Hypertension* 22 (2008). Full text:
http://www.nature.com/jhh/journal/v22/n6/full/1002311a.html

[5] Adriane Fugh-Berman, "Herbs and dietary supplement in the prevention and treatment of cardiovascular disease" *Preventative Cardiology* 3, (2000). Full text:
http://onlinelibrary.wiley.com/doi/10.1111/j.1520-037X.2000.80355.x/full

[6] GS Sonavane, et al., "Anxiogenic activity of Myristica fragrans seeds," *Pharmacology, Biochemistry and Behavior* 71, (2002). Abstract only:
http://www.ncbi.nlm.nih.gov/pubmed/11812528

The Flesh of Madre Cacao

Personal notes from Heidi Jarvis ND, MH, School of Natural Medicine, Herbs of Grace Dispensary, and Earth Pharmaceuticals

A Glossary of Herbalism

Nina Katz

Do you feel befuddled by all of those terms? Are you curious about what a menstruum might be, or a nervine? Wondering what the exact difference is between an infusion and a decoction? Or what it means to macerate? Read on; the herbalist lexicographer will reveal it all!

Adaptogen	n.	An herb that enhances one's ability to thrive despite stress. Eleuthero, or Siberian Ginseng *(Eleutherococcus senticosus)* is a well-known adaptogen.
Aerial *parts*	n. pl.	The parts of a plant that grow above ground. Stems, leaves, and flowers are all aerial parts, in contrast to roots and rhizomes.
Alterative	n.	An herb that restores the body to health gradually and sustainably by strengthening one or more of the body's systems, such as the digestive or lymphatic system, or one or more of the vital organs, such as the liver or kidneys. Burdock *(Arctium lappa)* is an alternative.
	adj.	Restoring health gradually, as by strengthening one or more of the body's systems or vital organs.
Anthel*mintic*	n.	A substance that eliminates intestinal worms.
Anthel*min*	adj.	Being of or concerning a substance that eliminates intestinal worms.
A*nti-cata*rrhal	n.	A substance that reduces or slows down the production of phlegm.
	adj.	Being of or concerning a substance that reduces or slows down the production of phlegm.
Anti-emetic	n.	A substance that treats nausea. Ginger *(Zingiber officinale)* is anti-emetic.
	adj.	Being of or concerning a substance that treats nausea.
Anti-mic*r*obial	n.	An herb or a preparation that helps the body fight

		off microbial infections, whether viral, bacterial, fungal, or parasitic. Herbal anti-microbials may do this by killing the microbes directly, but more often achieve this by enhancing immune function and helping the body to fight off disease and restore balance.
	adj.	Being of or concerning an herb or a preparation that helps the body fight off microbial infections.
Aperient	n.	A gentle laxative, such as seaweed, plantain seeds (Plantago spp.), or ripe bananas.
	adj.	Being of or concerning a gentle laxative.
Aphrodisiac	n.	A substance that enhances sexual interest or desire.
	adj.	Being of or relating to a substance that enhances sexual interest or desire.
Astringent	n.	A food, herb, or preparation that causes tissues to constrict, or draw in. Astringents help stop bleeding, diarrhea, and other conditions in which some bodily substance is flowing excessively. Some astringents, such as Wild Plantain (Plantago major), draw so powerfully that they can remove splinters.
	adj	Causing tissues to constrict, and thereby helping to stop excessive loss of body fluids.
Bitter	n.	A food, herb, or preparation that stimulates the liver and digestive organs through its bitter flavor. Dandelion (Taraxacum officinale) and Gentian (Gentiana lutea) are both bitters. Also called digestive bitter.
Carminative	n.	A food, herb, or preparation that reduces the buildup or facilitates the release of intestinal gases. Cardamom (Amomum spp. and Elettaria spp) and Fennel (Foeniculum vulgare) are carminatives.
	adj.	Characterized as reducing the buildup or facilitating the release of intestinal gases.

*Ca*rrier Oil	n.	A non-medicinal oil, such as olive or sesame oil, used to dilute an essential oil.
Ca*tarrh*	n.	An inflammation of the mucous membranes resulting in an overproduction of phlegm.
Com*pound*	v.	To create a medicinal formula using two or more components.
	n.	An herbal preparation consisting of two or more herbs.
*Com*press	n.	A topical preparation consisting of a cloth soaked in a liquid herbal extract, such as an infusion or decoction, and applied, usually warm or hot, to the body. A washcloth soaked in a hot ginger decoction and applied to a sore muscle is a compress.
De*coct*	v.	To prepare by simmering in water, usually for at least 20 minutes. One usually decocts barks, roots, *rhizomes*, hard seeds, twigs, and nuts.
De*coct*ion	n.	An herbal preparation made by simmering the plant parts in water, usually for at least 20 minutes.
De*mul*cent	n.	An herb with a smooth, slippery texture soothing to the mucous membranes, i.e. the tissues lining the respiratory and digestive tracts. Slippery elm *(Ulmus rubra)*, marshmallow root *(Althaea officinalis)*, and sassafras *(Sassafras albidum, Sassafras officinale)* are all demulcents.
	adj.	Having a smooth, slippery texture that soothes the mucous membranes.
Diapho*ret*ic	n.	An herb or preparation that opens the pores of the skin, facilitates sweat, and thereby lowers fevers. In Chinese medicine, diaphoretics are said to "release the exterior."□ Yarrow *(Achillea millefolium)* is a diaphoretic.
	adj.	Opening the pores, facilitating sweat, and thereby lowering fevers.
Di*ges*tive	n.	An herb, food, or preparation that promotes the healthy breakdown, assimilation, and elimination of food, as by gently stimulating the digestive tract

		in preparation for a meal. Dandelion *(Taraxacum officinale)* and bitter salad greens are digestives.
	adj. 1	Concerning or being part of the bodily system responsible for the breakdown, assimilation, and elimination of food.
	adj. 2	Promoting the healthy breakdown, assimilation, and/or elimination of food.
Diuretic	n.	A substance that facilitates or increases urination. Diuretics can improve kidney function and treat swelling. Excessive use of diuretics can also tax the kidneys. Stinging Nettles *(Urtica dioica)*, cucumbers, and coffee are all diuretics.
	adj.	Facilitating or increasing urination.
Emmenagogue	n.	An herb or preparation that facilitates or increases menstrual flow. Black cohosh *(Cimicifuga racemosa)* is an emmenagogue. Emmenagogues are generally contraindicated in pregnancy.
	adj.	Facilitating or increasing menstrual flow.
Essential *Oil*	n.	An oil characterized by a strong aroma, strong taste, the presence of terpines, and by vaporizing in low temperatures. Essential oils are components of many plants, and when isolated, make fairly strong medicine used primarily externally or for inhalation, and usually not safe for internal use.
	n. 1	A preparation made by chemically removing the soluble parts of a substance into a solvent or menstruum. Herbalists often make extracts using water, alcohol, glycerin, vinegar, oil, or combinations of these. Infusions, medicinal vinegars, tinctures, decoctions, and medicinal oils are all extracts.
	n. 2	A tincture.
Extract	v.	To remove the soluble parts of a substance into a solvent or menstruum by chemical means.
Febrifuge	n.	An herb or preparation that lowers fevers. Yarrow *(Achillea millefolium)*, ginger *(Zingiber officinale)*, and boneset *(Eupatorium perfoliatum)* are all febrifuges.
Galactagogue	n.	A substance that increases the production or flow of milk; a remedy that aids lactation. Nettle *(Urtica dioica)* and hops *(Humulus lupulus)* are

		galactagogues.
*Glan*dular	n.	A substance that treats the adrenal, thyroid, or other glands. Nettle seeds *(Urtica dioica)* are a glandular for the adrenals.
	adj.	Relating to or treating the adrenal, thyroid, or other glands.
He*pa*tic	n.	A substance that treats the liver. Dandelion *(Taraxacum officinale)* is a hepatic.
Hyp*n*otic	n.	An herb or preparation that induces sleep. Chamomile *(Matricaria recutita)* and valerian *(Valeriana officinale)* are both hypnotics.
	adj.	Inducing sleep.
In*fuse*	v.	To prepare by steeping in water, especially hot water, straining, and squeezing the marc.
In*fus*ion	n.	A preparation made by first steeping one or more plants or plant parts in water, most often hot water, and then straining the plant material, usually while squeezing the marc. An infusion extracts the flavor, aroma, and water-soluble nutritional and medicinal constituents into the water.
Long In*fus*ion	n.	An infusion that steeps for three or more hours. Long infusions often steep overnight.
Lym*ph*atic	n.	A substance that stimulates the circulation of lymph or *tonifies* the vessels or organs involved in the circulation or storage of lymph.
*Ma*cerate	v.	To soak a plant or plant parts in a *menstruum* so as to extract the medicinal constituents chemically.
Marc	n.	The plant material left after straining a preparation made by steeping, simmering, or macerating.
*Men*struum	n.	*(Plural, **menstrua** or **menstruums**.)* The solvent used to extract the medicinal and/or nutritional constituents from a plant. Water, alcohol, vinegar, and glycerin are among the more common menstrua.
*Mu*cilage	n.	A thick, slippery, *demulcent* substance produced by a plant or microorganism.

Muci*lag*inous	n.	Having or producing mucilage; *demulcent.* Okra, marshmallow root *(Althaea officinalis)*, sassafras *(Sassafras albidum, Sassafras officinale)*, and slippery elm *(Ulmus rubra)* are all mucilaginous.
*Nerv*ine	n.	An herb or preparation that helps with problems traditionally associated with the nerves, such as mental health issues, insomnia, and pain.
	adj.	Helping with problems traditionally associated with the nerves, such as mental health issues, insomnia, and pain.
Pectoral	n.	A substance that treats the lungs or the respiratory system.
*Poul*tice	n.	A mass of plant material or other substances, usually mashed, gnashed, moistened, or heated, and placed directly on the skin. Sometimes covered by a cloth or adhesive. A plantain *(Plantago spp.)* poultice can draw splinters out.
*Rhiz*ome	n.	A usually horizontal stem that grows underground, is marked by nodes from which roots grow down, and branches out to produce a network of new plants growing up from the nodes.
Salve	[sæv] n.	A soothing ointment prepared from beeswax combined with oil, usually medicinal oil, and used in topical applications.
Short Infusion	n.	An *infusion* that steeps for a relatively short period of time, usually 5-30 minutes.
Sedative	n.	A substance that calms and facilitates sleep. Valerian *(Valeriana officinale)* is a sedative.
Sedative	adj.	Calming and facilitating sleep.
*Sim*ple	n.	An herbal preparation, such as a tincture or decoction, made from one herb alone.
*Sim*pler	n.	An herbalist who prepares and recommends primarily *simples* rather than compounds.
Spp.	abbr. n.pl.	Species. *Used to indicate more than one species in the same botanical family. Echinacea spp.* includes both *Echinacea purpurea* and *Echinacea angustifolium*, among other species. *Plantago spp.*

		includes both *Plantago major* and *Plantago lanceolata*.
Stimulant	n.	An herb or preparation that increases the activity level in an organ or body system. Echinacea *(Echinacea spp.)* is an immunostimulant; it stimulates the immune system. Cayenne *(Capsicum spp.)* is a circulatory stimulant. Rosemary is a stimulant to the nervous, digestive, and circulatory systems.
Sudorific	adj.	Increasing sweat or facilitating the release of sweat; cf. *diaphoretic.*
Syrup	n.	A sweet liquid preparation, often made by adding honey or sugar to a decoction.
Tea	n.	A drink made by steeping a plant or plant parts, especially *Camellia sinensis.*
Tisane	n.	An herbal beverage made by decoction or short infusion and not prepared from the tea plant *(Camellia sinensis).*
Tincture	n.	A preparation made by macerating one or more plants or plant parts in a *menstruum,* usually alcohol or glycerin, straining, and squeezing the *marc* in order to extract the chemical constituents into the *menstruum.*
	v.	To prepare by *macerating* in a *menstruum,* straining, and squeezing the marc in order to extract the chemical constituents.
Tonic	n.	A substance that strengthens one or more organs or systems, or the entire organism. Stinging nettle *(Urtica dioica)* is a general tonic, as well as a specific kidney, liver, and hair tonic. Red raspberry leaf *(Rubus idaeus)* is a reproductive tonic; Mullein *(Verbascum thapsus)* is a respiratory tonic.
Tonify	v.	To strengthen. Nettle *(Urtica dioica)* tonifies the entire body.
Volatile Oil	n.	An oil characterized by volatility, or rapid vaporization at relatively low temperatures; cf. *essential oil.*
Vulnerary	n.	A substance that soothes and heals wounds. Comfrey *(Symphytum officinale)* is an excellent vulnerary.
	adj.	Being or concerning a substance that soothes and heals wounds.

Disclaimer

Nothing provided by Natural Living Mamma LLC, Natural Herbal Living Magazine, or Herb Box should be considered medical advice. Nothing included here is approved by the FDA and the information provided herein is for informational purposes only. Always consult a botanically knowledgeable medical practitioner before starting any course of treatment, especially if you are pregnant, breastfeeding, on any medications, or have any health problems. Natural Living Mamma LLC is not liable for any action or inaction you take based on the information provided here.

Made in the USA
Middletown, DE
28 February 2023

25907422R00024